10/3
X 10/10

One in Four: Shifting the Balance on Pregnancy Loss

Barbara Toppin, M.D.

One in Four

Shifting the Balance on Pregnancy Loss

© 2013 Barbara Toppin, M.D.

This book is designed to promote greater understanding of reproductive and pregnancy health for interested readers. Its content is the sole expression and opinion of its author. No guaranteed outcomes are expressed or implied by the author's choice to include any of the content in this book. This book and its contents are not intended to take the place of medical advice from a trained medical professional. Please seek the advice of your medical care provider before trying any new treatment. Neither the publisher nor the author shall be liable for any physical, psychological, emotional, financial, or commercial damages, including, but not limited to, special, incidental, consequential or other damages. You are responsible for the actions you choose to take, and for their results.

ISBN 978-1482728903

To all the future parents and families.

One in Four: Shifting the Balance on Pregnancy Loss

Introduction

New Paradigms for Pregnancy Health

My Story

As an ObGyn, I had always been certain my body would never betray me in my desire for a child. Yet by the time my husband and I were ready to conceive, I was 40 years old, and I knew it was unlikely my story would be as straightforward as I had hoped. We had met later in our lives, and spent our younger years as so many do today, entirely absorbed in building our respective careers. Delayed childbearing was a necessary but unfortunate consequence of that dedication to learning our trades.

At 40—and at the edge of reasonably attempting to get pregnant on our own—we only tried "the fun way" for about three months. Certain that an infertility specialist would be able to help, we eagerly made an appointment to begin this new phase of our life, family, and relationship. Yet what I encountered in our initial physician meeting was a rote, cookbook approach to fertility medicine: a few months of fertility drugs followed by intrauterine insemination, and—if we could afford it—in vitro fertilization.

To make matters worse, I was offered no explanation for my infertility other than that I simply had "old eggs". Moreover, my age would limit me to the option of carrying a donor egg in vitro. Without many choices, we decided to try the fertility drugs and intrauterine insemination, but had no success. After two years of attempts, we finally made the painful decision to stop trying to conceive in 2002.

Had I known what I know today about thrombophilias (disorders that promote blood clotting) and their effects on pregnancy loss, many of the dangers I faced when seeking to conceive would have been eliminated. Instead, my husband and I resolved ourselves to not having children. I eagerly turned my thoughts toward the private practice I had just joined, and the task of helping my patients conceive and maintain healthy pregnancies themselves.

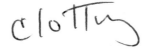
clotting

As my private practice in Minnesota grew, I encountered new enthusiasm for studying and learning all I could about conception and pregnancy loss. Observing my patients, I noticed that many of them had challenges with blood clotting disorders, called thrombophilias. But the turning point did not come until 2004, when I attended my first online conference with perinatologists on the topic of clotting disorders.

Sheer curiosity led me to join the seminar, and I listened with rapt attention to the lectures and questions regarding thrombophilia and pregnancy loss. A world of information opened up before me, and I immediately began wondering how this information might benefit the patients I treat who experience recurrent loss. Inspired by the work of Drs. Andrzej Petryk and Majed Abu-Hajir, who began the first pregnancy and coagulation clinic in the country, my medical partner Dr. Wanda Adefris and I began developing a methodology to incorporate this approach into our patient care.

Our very first patient was a woman who had in vitro fertilization four times prior, and was on the verge of filing to adopt. I decided to offer her the new information I had obtained, and she was interested in exploring its relevance to her situation. Testing her for evidence of thrombophilia, we discovered that she did have a genetic tendency to blood clotting. We then treated her for this potentiality, and she subsequently was able to have four babies under our care. Dr. Adefris and I could not have been more thrilled.

Once I saw the positive effects of this treatment, I began looking back at my own family history and the challenges I had becoming pregnant. I was astonished to discover the medical challenges my family faced. We had it all: An unexplained heart attack in a sister at age 46, prematurity (pre-term births), colon cancer, and even cerebral palsy. Ironically, an aspirin or Heparin (the most common treatment for basic thrombophilia) might have helped me to conceive.

Thrombophilia works forward and backward, as you can look at a family history and predict certain medical events an individual may face. In this way, prevention of problems in pregnancy hinges in part on my ability as a physician to interpret my patients' personal and family histories. Looking forward, knowing that an individual has a thrombophilia may prevent a pregnancy loss, a stroke, a heart attack, and/or a fatal event related to these problems. Knowing what I now know not only provides the relief of an explanation for the pain of pregnancy loss, but, more importantly, allows the individual to prevent needless future suffering.

Today, I am committed to giving this opportunity for understanding and possible prevention of pregnancy loss to every patient I see. I know that I cannot prevent all disease, but I would like to see a more thoughtful approach to medicine that applies generous but equal portions of logic, intuition, compassion, and common sense alongside evidence-based medicine.

The Possibility of Hope

A patient I'll call Amanda was 30 years old when she came to my office. She seemed to be a very quiet and anxious woman who spoke only when asked a question. After obtaining her history, I found out that she had suffered two previous pregnancy losses. The first was a spontaneous loss at 18 weeks, and the second was a more devastating loss of an anencephalic baby at 20 weeks. Anencephaly is a defect of the formation of the neural tube associated with deficient amounts of folic acid, preventing the fetal skull and brain from forming. Amanda's former doctor suggested she continue trying to maintain a healthy pregnancy without the benefit of any testing or counseling. She had an absolute fear of becoming pregnant again, and was on the verge of giving up on the idea of having her own biologic child until a group of concerned friends stepped in. These women gave her my name, and, with some gentle coaxing over several months, she made an appointment.

During the course of my evaluation, I found that Amanda had a genetic disorder called MTHFR-C677T, which interferes with the metabolism of folic acid. Folic acid is needed for cell growth and fetal development. Inability to process folate may also cause an increased risk of blood clots. Suddenly, we had one potential answer to the question of why she had suffered two very different losses. I informed Amanda of the problem and together we made a plan of action. I explained that our approach was unique to what other doctors might try, and immediately sensed her apprehension and lack of trust for physicians and medicine. This hesitancy filled me with determination to gain her confidence, as I knew I would not have a second chance.

We started administering extra folate and treated Amanda with an injectable anticoagulant. She dutifully learned to inject herself, took her folate, and never missed a visit. Amanda would enter the room quietly and answer my questions precisely yet without much emotion. She had no questions of her own, and was reticent to say more than a few words. I was delighted as the pregnancy passed the gestational age of her first loss, but got no feedback—positive or negative—from Amanda.

3

The next significant event was the level II sonogram. Normally we perform ultrasounds in our office, but due to her history of having an anencephalic baby, Amanda needed to have her 20-week scan with a perinatologist. Although I was confident that the fetus would be normal, as she had had normal scans at 8 and 12 weeks, my staff and I held our collective breath when the day arrived.

Spontaneous cheers broke when we heard the news—a normal and healthy baby boy! I expected that the mother would finally show signs of excitement or happiness, but found that neither she nor her husband would allow themselves to express anything more than a flat and fearful demeanor. Time passed, she felt fetal kicks and movements, and we saw perfect growth and development of the baby. Still, there were no signs that she was reassured by what was happening.

I tried to get Amanda to talk about her fears and feelings but could not get through. I knew that she would have followed any instructions I gave her without question, but her affect was entirely flat. I worried about the potential of depression, but she denied any symptoms. Her problem was sheer terror.

To say that our staff pampered her would be an understatement. Our team is filled with dedicated doctors, nurses, assistants, and business staff, all prepared for handholding whenever needed. We watched her baby grow and supported her and her husband for the entirety of the pregnancy. The day of her delivery arrived, and I watched with great hope as her labor progressed normally. Still, Amanda's fear was palpable. She gently pushed her baby boy into the world, and I placed him on her chest.

A few silent tears filled her eyes as she and her husband marveled at their son. They entered their own world of bonding and wonder: She felt no pain as the placenta was delivered, did not release the baby to the nurse to be weighed, and barely heard my congratulations. I could not have been happier.

About two years later, Amanda returned for her next pregnancy. I entered the exam room expecting to find the woman I knew prior. Yet in the place of the quiet, fearful patient I expected, I found a person full of life and conversation. She told me how she had begun planning her second pregnancy by calling our staff to start the needed medication at the appropriate time. She knew her "formula," and over the next nine months followed it perfectly, buoyed by a newfound confidence and spirit.

Since that time, I have seen numerous other patients transform from helpless, sad, and fearful women to self-assured mothers who know that they are not at the mercy of nature and genetics.

Confronting Pregnancy Loss

While loss of a pregnancy is always a devastating event for a woman and those close to her, physicians often discount early losses as non-events, treating the fetus as a non-entity. Moreover, miscarriage is rarely discussed between patient and physician prior to a pregnancy; it is a dark secret, whispered sympathetically only after the loss has already occurred. It is then that physicians, family members, and other women sadly come forth to share their stories.

Grief and fear commingle equally at such a time, a heavy emotional burden increased by a lack of knowledge regarding the underlying causes of the loss. Without understanding, fear of recurring loss will perpetuate, leading to anxiety about never having a baby—and feeding the looming fear of failure.

This book aims to create a sphere of influence in reproductive medicine, extending beyond the women I have encountered in my 26 years of practice as an ObGyn. Its content is intended to educate and inspire women who want to reclaim health and power in their reproductive process. As much as I write for patients, I also hope healthcare providers will find equal value in these pages. Ideally, the book will establish a platform for thoughtful discussion about recurrent pregnancy loss and prevention. This book is not meant to be the ultimate guide on the subject of reproductive health, nor should it become an obstacle to good care.

Of course, our approach can and will continue to improve. I have one patient who has had many losses in spite of our combined best efforts. She has faith in our investigations and knows that I will support her throughout the process as we seek advice from other forward thinking specialists. Together, we look for answers and make changes to her care as indicated. Through our investigations, we discovered some medical conditions that needed attention, and this patient now has an excellent understanding of the events surrounding her losses. Remarkably, she lives a wonderfully full and balanced life, maintaining a positive attitude supported by the understanding that I stand with her and her family.

It is my hope that all women feel not only the support of their doctors during times of loss, but the hope that comes from being able to obtain answers and make changes in the future.

Acknowledging and investigating the loss will provide the family with critical options, including the choice to try again equipped with greater knowledge about their unique genetic infrastructure. The information that we learn from our losses is important to the mother, her future children, and the entire family.

Most importantly, I want to inspire women to become actively involved with their own healthcare, and to overcome the fears surrounding the loss of a baby by equipping themselves with knowledge about their own bodies in order to move forward confidently. Furthermore, I want to show that through exploration and treatment of some of the common causes of miscarriage, women and their families may be positively affected with longer, healthier lives.

The information in this book will continue to change and improve as medical research seeks an innovative edge to reproductive health. I hope that my colleagues and I will continue to strive to deliver the most optimal and personalized care to our patients as the field evolves.

Chapter One

An Unacceptable Statistic

> Penance need not be paid in suffering...It can be paid in forward motion. Correcting the mistake is a positive move, a nurturing move.
> — Barbara Hall —

The statistics on pregnancy loss, prematurity, and other complications of pregnancy in the U.S. are simply not acceptable. The country boasts an absurdly high 1 in 4 miscarriage rate, and the maternal death rate in the U.S. is 17/100,000 women. In Croatia it is 14/100.000, and in Italy it is only 4/100,000.

In all pregnancies, there is a 10-15% risk of miscarriage, which may actually be as high as 20-25% because of unrecognized, ultra-early losses. The risk increases to 20% in women who have had a previous loss. This percentage rises with age (10-17% for ages 20-30, 20-33% for ages 30-35, 40% up to age 40, and 80% for those over 44). The age differential is linked to possible poor quality of eggs, which may not be compatible with life and/or lead to chromosomal problems in the baby. With recent studies suggesting that a large majority of eggs may be lost by age 30, miscarriage statistics have been compounded by intervals of infertility.

Unfortunately, these statistics are taught in medical school and accepted as sad but true facts that we can do nothing about. We have been taught that no investigation is needed when a first or second pregnancy is lost. It would be unthinkable to ask a person who has suffered a stroke, heart attack, or a cancerous tumor to wait until they have had 3 related incidents before any investigation occurred. Yet modern medicine asks women and their families to wait until they have had 2 or 3 miscarriages before seeking to address the underlying causes, as if it were a trivial complication. Change to this dogma, in general, is very slow to come.

This first struck me as unacceptable during my residency 20 years ago, when I was rotating within a very affluent private hospital in New Jersey. As a junior resident, I was responsible for admitting patients who were due to have surgery the next day. There, I met a 38-year-old woman who was admitted for a tubal sterilization. In taking her history, I saw that she had had 6 prior pregnancies, and no living children. When I asked her about this, she explained that she had lost each of those pregnancies early, the earliest at 6 weeks, and the latest at 16. I was shocked that she was now choosing to have a sterilization, removing any future possibility of pregnancy. She began to sob, telling me that she no longer had the heart to try again.

This patient had been worked up with tests for infection and a sonogram to assess her uterus for abnormalities and was told that there was no apparent reason for her losses. Soon after, she gave up hope and chose what seemed to be the only option to end her suffering—sterilization. I tried to inspire her to seek other advice, but her doctor assured her that "everything" had been done to help her, and her situation was simply one of those great "unknowns." There was nothing I could do to change her mind.

Although this woman went through with the procedure, I never forgot her. Two decades have passed since then, but patients today are similarly given a bereavement booklet, instructed to try again, and sent on their way to suffer in fear and silence. While it may not be as evident, healthcare providers also suffer in the face of pregnancy loss, as they grapple with their own inability to answer their patients' ultimate question: *Why did this happen to me?*

Most physicians believe that the next pregnancy will be fine, and for many women it is. Other families will suffer recurrent losses, but are offered no solutions other than to keep trying. Some physicians will perform a limited testing of the products of conception that were miscarried if available, but most simply follow the doctrine of the medical text, dictating that no workup is needed until the patient has 3 or more miscarriages. Much of obstetrics is still practiced this way, either due to a rigid adherence to medical dogma, an attempt to honor financial considerations like insurance coverage, or just because no better way is known.

The by-the-book method seems a safe bet because many subsequent pregnancies will result in a healthy baby. Yet this method fails to consider the many other pregnancy complications suffered by those who have "healthy" babies. In addition, it does not address the patients who have losses in later trimesters. Moreover, this approach entirely ignores the 20% of women who will repeat a pregnancy loss.

Yet this medical doctrine was written over 40 years ago, for a different group of women who had babies at much younger ages and had a longer span of their fertile lives to work with. This philosophy and approach never evolved to meet the needs of today's woman. Planning a family in this century may start after age 25 and go well into a woman's thirties.

New data show that a maternal genetic predisposition to thrombophilias such as Factor V Leiden and MTHFR can cause many pregnancy complications, including both early and late pregnancy losses. The good news is that these predispositions can be fairly easy to treat and may provide insight into potential future health problems, like heart attacks, stokes, blood clotting disorders and even colon cancer. Genetic causes of pregnancy loss seem to "turn on" in the late 20's, and may coincide with a woman's first pregnancy, resulting in disaster.

Why is this so unacceptable? The answer is simple, and no great secret: Many of these losses and complications are preventable. This guide does not seek to put you at odds with your physician, nor does it seek to dictate my method as the only way. It is merely an outline to give new options to those who have suffered a pregnancy loss.

Today, I know that I could have helped the woman who chose sterilization 20 years ago in New Jersey. Had we been able to initiate a workup with the first loss, or before, and aggressively test for thrombophilias, autoimmune disorders, and genetic, medical and anatomic reasons for miscarriage, we may have been able to get to the root of the problem and prevent recurrent loss. With her in mind, I seek to offer every patient the most complete and realistic approach to her pregnancy and reproductive health.

Chapter 1: An Unacceptable Statistic

Many pregnancy losses are unacceptable.

Many pregnancy losses are preventable.

Some causes of pregnancy loss are genetic in nature.

Some of the genetic causes may imply that a woman is predisposed to future medical problems like heart attacks, strokes, blood clots and colon cancer.

Chapter Two

Making Sense of Suffering

If you have a wonderful truth to tell, rarely will you be believed.
— The Alchemist, Paul Coelho —

Suffering never makes sense to me, and as a doctor, I am committed to presenting my patients with information that makes real sense. Suffering may serve a purpose in medicine, but only when it leads to information that lends itself to discovering a healthier life. Suffering one miscarriage is bad enough; waiting for 3 before anything is done to investigate the underlying causes is outrageous.

Pregnancy Loss by "The Book"

More than 40 years ago, the norm was for women to marry young and start their families in their late teens to early twenties. Women did not often wait to conceive until the third or fourth decades of life. Those who did have children at the age of 30 or higher were considered "elderly". Doctors viewed these patients with caution, and were correct to do so.

In these older women, they expected pregnancies complicated by early and late losses, toxemia, diabetes, and a myriad of other potential medical problems. When these women had losses, they were told that the cause of the miscarriage was chromosomal 50% of the time, infections 25% of the time, and entirely unknown 25% of the time. Patients were simply encouraged to try again, without any further investigation. The only way they participated in their own care was when they were placed on bed and pelvic rest for the next pregnancy, while everyone around them waited anxiously and hoped for the best.

If a subsequent loss occurred, the process was repeated. Only after the third or fourth loss was a very limited workup performed. Chromosome testing was done, infections were ruled out, and dye studies conducted to make sure there were no uterine abnormalities. After the third miscarriage, women often grew frustrated, desperate, and helpless. Many providers, disheartened by repeated failures, had a hard time facing the families. With nothing more to offer their patients after multiple losses, providers would grow distant and give up.

Patients then blamed themselves for imagined violations of the "rules" of pregnancy, often feeling that they deserved the loss. Far worse, some providers exhibited a willful ignorance of potential remedies for pregnancy loss, refusing to explore or investigate in spite of patient requests or suggestions from consultants (such as perinatologists, who often empirically suggest treating for thrombophilia after 3 or more losses).

If women were able to make it out of the first trimester, they were usually overwhelmed with fear for the remainder of their pregnancy. Many of those pregnancies were troubled and complicated by growth retardation toxemia, preterm labor, and even full-term demise. Although decades have passed since the scenarios I describe here, much remains the same in the realm of managing pregnancy loss.

Causes of Miscarriage

In my own practice, I have the privilege of caring for many patients who have faced numerous pregnancy losses without any significant action taken to discern the underlying causes of these complications. I recently spoke with one patient who had 3 losses without a workup and was on the verge of tubal sterilization. Fortunately, I gained her confidence by discussing her options, and she allowed one more trial. I can happily report that she has had two children since then, and recently decided to complete her sterilization.

A simple workup for her revealed a tendency to thrombophilias, which we treated effectively with a blood thinner. We monitored her babies throughout both pregnancies, looking for subtle changes in the blood flow resistance in the umbilical arteries, and rapid aging of the placenta, which would affect the baby's growth. She delivered without complications, and because of her blood-clotting tendency, she is now cognizant of potential problems with birth control pills, hormonal replacement, and other forms of hormonal contraception.

There is no rule stating that a patient must have only one cause of pregnancy loss. One of our very brave patients had 12 pregnancies by the age of 35, having started in her early 20s. She had seen many physicians, and after having 4 losses, was finally worked up. Her husband was found to have had a balanced translocation of chromosomes. This is an abnormality where a small amount of a chromosome changes places with the same amount of genetic material from another chromosome. Although frustrating, she was very glad at least to know what the cause was. She knew that one of 4 or 5 pregnancies could be successful, and was eventually able to have one full term pregnancy.

This patient spent her own money for in vitro fertilization and traveled to other states for the in vitro procedure. She came to our clinic because of frustrations with her prior physicians. Reviewing what had been done to investigate the losses, we found she had not been thoroughly tested. A blood test showed that she had a thrombophilias tendency, adding to the challenge of the chromosomal abnormality. Although many of the losses were due to the abnormal chromosomes or gene, some may have been due to an inherited clotting disorder. We treated her with Heparin beginning with ovulation during her subsequent cycle, as she was simultaneously undergoing in vitro fertilization. She successfully conceived twins that were delivered at term. When she tried again, however, she had many more losses.

Another patient presented with 7 pregnancy losses. When asked what was done to work her up, she replied that she had been told they did not know why she kept losing the pregnancies, and to just keep trying. This patient had insulin dependent diabetes, yet was never advised that she needed a complete thrombophilia and thyroid workup prior to getting pregnant. Our evaluation revealed a thyroid condition, for which we began treatment. She began taking thyroid medication and Heparin before her next conception, and was subsequently able to have two children.

Moreover, many women present for what they consider to be difficulty conceiving. Because of this, a miscarriage may go unrecognized by the patient and provider without careful discernment of those presenting with infertility.

One patient reported that she felt the symptoms of early pregnancy almost every month for an entire year. She had been charting her temperature graphs and doing ovulation testing and she seemed to be ovulating. She had breast tenderness and extreme fatigue. Each month her hopes were high, yet she would routinely have her menses a day or two late and slightly heavier than what she had normally experienced. She was so convinced that she was pregnant each month that she preformed regular urine pregnancy tests, all of which returned negative.

13

She began the infertility workup at our clinic, and was asked to have a progesterone level test and come in for a blood pregnancy test when she missed her period. The following month, her progesterone level was normal and she had a negative urine pregnancy test. Although a blood pregnancy test returned positive, she had her menses the following day. It grew apparent that she was having losses so early that they were barely perceptible.

These cases demonstrate the range of challenges faced by couples seeking healthy pregnancy—and the broad spectrum of treatment possibilities. Allowing anyone to continue to have pregnancy loss makes no sense. Providers need to approach the problem of loss in the most efficient and caring manner, which includes a more thorough and aggressive stance to determine the unique physiological and genetic challenges each woman faces in her progress towards a healthy pregnancy and birth.

Nothing gives me greater pleasure than telling a couple that I can help them. A workup is done for couples presenting with infertility, one pregnancy loss, and for those at risk who are presenting for pre-pregnancy planning. Although this method does not always work, at this writing I have only 2 patients (out of the hundreds I treat each year) who present with recurrent losses in spite of our best efforts. These women remain my patients because they are aware that our hearts and minds are open to learning about their unique situations and treating them with the resulting insights. I am hopeful that together we can make sensible decisions regarding the right approach.

As described in the following chapters on workup and treatments, a creative thought process is needed to help those couples with the most challenging problems. This approach eschews the traditional medical doctrine in order to provide individualized medical solutions that deliver true possibilities for pregnancy health.

Chapter 2: Making Sense of Suffering

15-25% of pregnancies will end in miscarriage; the old rule of allowing 3 losses before investigating no longer applies.

Pregnancy loss may be multifactorial, and must be addressed on an individual, personalized, and exhaustive basis of inquiry, analysis, and treatment.

Chapter Three

The Workup

Don't despise empiric truth. Lots of things work in practice for which the laboratory has never found proof.
— Martin H. Fischer —

What does a workup for pregnancy loss involve? Unfortunately there is no definitive answer. I can only give my suggested workup, which covers a wide range of potential problems. Ideally, in order to prevent losses and suffering, most of this information should be obtained when women are considering pregnancy for the first time. Many of my patients, however, arrive for their first prenatal visit only to discover that the fetal heart tone is no longer present. After delivering this devastating news and giving the patient the time they need to grieve, we always investigate options for a workup and make plans for future treatments.

Recently, a 26 year-old former patient visited me for consultation after she had moved 3 hours away. She originally presented to my office at the age of 23 with a deep venous thrombosis in her leg while planning a pregnancy and currently on birth control pills. With the history of a known cardiovascular event, I worked her up, performing a detailed history, physical, and lab testing, as I would for anyone who had had a previous pregnancy loss.

A thrombophilia of the A mutation of MTHFR was revealed. Ordinarily, I would have treated her with a children's aspirin, however our hematologist and I felt that treatment with Lovenox was warranted due to the previous blood clot. Her pregnancy was uncomplicated and she had a full term delivery. A few years later, the patient told me that she was moving away. My office provided her with her records and advice that she should take Heparin for all subsequent pregnancies to prevent early loss and other morbidities associated with thrombophilias.

When she presented to me 3 years after her move, she was very upset. She had sought care with an obstetrician closer to home, but recently had a miscarriage at 9 weeks. She had discussed her previous blood clot with her physician and was told that she did not need anticoagulation therapy in spite of reviewing our records. During a routine dating sonogram, a fetal demise of the pregnancy was diagnosed.

Although we never knew the cause of the loss, my patient understood that she would have increased her chances of a successful pregnancy by following her previous treatment path. We discussed her options, and as I reviewed my previous records, I was startled to find that she was only heterozygous for the A mutation, which did not usually cause severe effects. Since her last pregnancy, I had learned that people who were heterozygous for the A mutation seemed to have milder side effects and were effectively treated with children's aspirin.

Yet the overarching question was why this patient had had a blood clot at such a young age. She had no other risk factors, such as smoking or obesity. Over the course of the years she had moved away, I also learned of two new tests for thrombophilias, separate from the MTHFR, and tested her. She had a lipoprotein level that was higher than any I had ever seen. That gave me a more definite diagnosis, and again supported what the patient and I both intuitively knew. She is planning another pregnancy and will take Lovenox.

Medicine is dynamic, but our genetic predispositions are not. If someone has had a previous blood clot they are likely to have another. If anything, those predispositions may be expressed even more strongly with normal aging. At the same time, many providers feel that performing a few tests covers all bases and assures that a patient's condition will remain static over time.

If I have learned nothing else from talking to patients it is this: Everything has not **ever** been done. There are no definitives in medicine, and all providers have their own ideas on how to treat their patients. The best we can do is provide suggestions of what has worked for the majority of our patients.

Personal History

All medical providers have been taught to obtain a medical history, yet many of the clues to the ultimate cause of miscarriage contained in that history are often overlooked.

Some of the clues I use are as follows.

Physical Exam

General physical and gynecologic exams will help to eliminate the possibility of obvious congenital (birth condition) problems. There are many physical and mental conditions that need to be addressed prior to undergoing any course of treatment. Simply taking a blood pressure or pulse may reveal underlying conditions that can easily be corrected.

Pregnancy History

How many other pregnancies have you had and at what age did you have them? Was there a history of low birth weight or premature labor? If you had a PENTA screen, was there a false positive report? Were there any comments on the placenta? Have you been told that you had a placental abruption, DIC, or that you had heavy bleeding? Have you had early cervical dilation?

Menstrual History

How often do you have your menses? How long are they? What is the interval between cycles? Are they painful? Do you have large clots? Does your pain come halfway through your cycle? Do you have significant pain with bowel movements or urination?

Gynecologic History

Have you had STDs? Abnormal Pap smears, colposcopy, a LEEP procedure, or a cone biopsy?

Previous Pregnancy Losses

This will include the number and description of any losses, any chromosomal abnormalities, loss presentation; bleeding or on sonogram; sac or fetus size in comparison to dates; comparative dates of loss in recurrent losses; ectopic or molar pregnancies; and stillbirths.

Medical Conditions

Heart disease, diabetes, hypertension, thyroid disease, migraines, allergies, polycystic ovary syndrome, endometriosis, autoimmune diseases history of infertility, psychoemotional problems, depression and anxiety, and bleeding or clotting tendencies are all significant factors.

Surgical History

Surgical history including laparoscopy, cesarean, D&C, as well as surgical complications and related conditions such as smoking, drugs, and alcohol usage.

Family History

Family history of heart disease (heart attack, stroke, pulmonary embolism, blood clots), diabetes, colon cancer, and unusual cancers (like lung cancer in people without a history of smoking exposure). Are your parents and grandparents alive? If not, from what did they die? Are there any people with cerebral palsy, or unknown causes of mental retardation, in your family. Any early deaths?

My favorite question is: *Are your parents and siblings all alive?* This helps me find medical conditions that most people do not associate with pregnancy loss. It also identifies conditions in terms that the patient and family understand. For instance, hypertension may be called high blood pressure, or diabetes called "sugar diabetes". It is very important that we all speak the same language.

Are you adopted? This presents a special challenge. If little or no information is known about a person's family history, I perform a complete lab workup.

Social History

Do you smoke? Do you use drugs? Drink alcohol? History of abuse?
Are you safe now?

Lab Workup

Lab exams may uncover hidden potential concerns that could not only help treat the problem of pregnancy loss but may also provide great insight into prevention of future problems.

I have divided the lab workup up into cultures and viral titer, blood, and radiological portions.

Cervical cultures may provide a simple answer to some fertility and pregnancy loss problems. These may include unusual problems that arise from communicable diseases, which may often be asymptomatic. Ideally these tests are preformed prior to a patient's pregnancy, based upon the history alone so that she may never suffer a loss. If I believe there may be a substantial risk of complications, I do draw them while she is pregnant. If the patient has had a loss, I usually wait until the miscarriage is complete and she has a negative HCG level before drawing the test, as some tests may be abnormal because of the loss.

What follows is the story of how a simple urine or vaginal culture can help reveal otherwise asymptomatic problems that may interfere with the pregnancy. A new patient of mine presented with a history of primary infertility, for which we conducted an infertility workup. After one cycle of treatment with clomiphene citrate, she conceived. Part of our prenatal lab profile included a routine urine culture, which revealed a bladder infection. Our patient was informed of our findings and given a prescription for amoxicillin at about 10 weeks pregnant.

One week later she presented to the emergency room with acute back pain, fever, lower abdominal cramping, and vaginal spotting. We did an ultrasound that showed a small bleed near the uterine sac, and also diagnosed her with acute pyelonephritis, a kidney infection. We then learned that the patient had not taken the prescribed antibiotics because she had not had any symptoms and did not feel it was needed. She was subsequently admitted to the hospital and treated with intravenous antibiotics.

Although her urine culture cleared up, she did not seem to respond well. Within a few days she was unable to walk or stand, and was in excruciating pain. An MRI showed an internal abscess involving her back and pelvic muscles. This woman remained in the hospital for most of her pregnancy and ultimately delivered at 37 weeks. The abscess was tested after she delivered and contained tuberculosis. She had lived in another country in the past and had pelvic TB. The urinary infection had been coincidental.

The labs I may obtain are dependent on individual patient presentation. Not every lab listed below is needed for every patient. Most importantly, I always make a plan of action when tests are ordered so that the next step in treatment is known prior to getting the test results.

Cultures and Viral Labs

Ureaplasm
Mycoplasm
STD cultures
Group B strep
Urine analysis
Urine culture
HPV
TORCH titers (rubella, rubeola, varicella cytomegalic hepatitis and parvo viruses)

Coagulation Labs

MTHFR
Factor V Leiden
PAI
Lipoprotein A
ANA
CBC (complete blood count)
Antithrombin
Protein S and C
Lupus anticoagulant
Homocysteine
Prothrombin
Anti beta 2 glycoprotein antibodies
Platelet count

Hormonal Labs

FSH
LH
Progesterone
TSH

Miscellaneous Labs

Chromosomes studies both partners
Semen analysis
Fragile X

Placental pathology
Autopsy
Chromosomes studies of miscarriage

Radiologic and Ultrasonic Testing
Pelvic sonogram
Sonohysterogram
Hysterosalpingogram

Group therapy and psychological support
Bereavement counseling
Group therapy
Family therapy

As new advances in medicine occur, there are always new tests to aid in the investigation of pregnancy loss. The lists above contain basic tests I have found helpful. Once I have the basic test results, I arrange for appropriate consultations as needed, such as referral to a hematologist or endocrinologist where additional testing may be performed as needed.

Chapter 3: The Workup

The possibility of loss is lessened if a workup is performed during preconception, prior to pregnancy.

A detailed history is needed to provide vital clues to possible reasons for pregnancy loss.

A broad spectrum of tests is needed to avoid too narrow a focus on a single suspected problem.

Chapter 4

Approaching Loss

A person cannot do great things; a person can only do small things with great love.
— Mother Theresa —

Early detection of a viable or nonviable pregnancy is the key to preventing future loss. Prior to the now ubiquitous office ultrasound machine, women who presented without fetal heart tones in the first and early second trimester were told that they would most likely hear them on the next visit. This is still practiced by many providers, yet provides no reassurance for the patient.

It is simply unacceptable not to hear the fetal heart tones at the first prenatal visit. Early identification of a loss is essential. The reasons are multiple, ranging from the immediate concerns for the pregnancy and fetus to the mother's longer-term health.

Of immediate concern are the dangers associated with various complications to pregnancy. While a large gestational sac or fetus may require surgical intervention such as a D&C, some women may face severe hemorrhage. Ectopic or tubal pregnancies must be identified and treated as early as possible. This may allow for non-surgical treatment and also prevent rupture, a potentially life-threatening condition.

Finally, one of the most important reasons for early detection is the mental health of the family. Once we have identified a fetal demise, we gently give the news to the patient. The reasons for the diagnosis are discussed and we honestly document the absence of the fetus or fetal heart tones, along with any observed abnormalities. We also try to give supportive care through our own capacities and suggestions for bereavement counseling as necessary, as it is hard information to share and take in. We try to dispel any guilty thoughts that may run through the minds of our patients, as many quickly turn to blame themselves. Most importantly, we allow them to grieve.

A second visit is then offered, and may be necessary for those with very early losses when there is any question of viability on either the part of the family or physician. When the family is ready, the possible reasons for the loss are discussed. The workup is not usually done until the patient is no longer pregnant, because some of the labs may be artificially abnormal due to the demise. Additional visits may be necessary to explain results of testing and to offer answers when possible.

Finally, we discuss the options for managing the current loss. Individual patient desires are addressed. If a sac is 6-7 weeks or under, there is no definitive rule to perform a D&C. It is likely that a woman may experience heavy bleeding for a few hours; she may also pass a small amount of tissue. These are both very common. We do ask the patient to come to the emergency room if she feels at all uncomfortable or if the bleeding is very heavy.

If the gestational sac or fetus is larger than measured at 7-8 weeks, it may be better to have a D&C, since heavy bleeding and moderate to severe pain is more likely and may occur at any time. Our patient may find herself needing emergent care, such as a blood transfusion. For miscarriages later than 12-14 weeks, induction of labor is usually needed. We typically use Misoprostil and Prostaglandin, which help to ripen the cervix and stimulate contractions. Second and third trimester losses will also need induction of labor. A D&C may also be chosen because the tissue can be examined for chromosomal and other potential causes of the miscarriage.

On rare occasions with a larger fetus, a D&E (dilation and evacuation) will be performed. This is potentially more hazardous because of the risks of perforation of the uterus by fetal bone tissue. A D&E is a process that is best performed when the benefits to the patient outweigh the risks. One of those conditions is disseminated intravascular coagulation (DIC), which presents a very real risk of maternal death and may be seen when a larger fetus has been deceased for more than a few days or weeks.

Every patient has different thoughts on how to end a pregnancy that is no longer viable. We try to provide suggestions and supportive care that reflect the specific needs of each woman we treat. My desire is always to give hope for future pregnancies while acknowledging the challenges of the current pregnancy. For some, bereavement counselors are needed, while for others, simply allowing them to speak to other families who have had similar experiences may be helpful. Grief is a necessary emotion to address in whatever way is most conducive to the mother and her family's emotional makeup and wellbeing.

Providers must acknowledge the loss and not act as if nothing important has occurred. Patients should also understand that most providers are profoundly affected by the family's loss. They often feel a deep discomfort when dealing with grief, as most are taught to distance themselves from feelings of helplessness and fear for the patient. As my own mother was a nurse, I learned from a young age to listen to others with an openness to learning from them. This approach helps me lead with compassion, supporting my patients through moments that are often unspeakably difficult. In this way, bereavement is a necessary journey for both patient and provider.

I always make sure to explain that although future pregnancy is likely, the family is encouraged to take the time they need to heal emotionally. In spite of the best effort made to prevent a recurrence, another loss is always a possibility. The patient and her family need to be able to endure the pressures and fears associated with the next pregnancy. There is no set timeframe for grief; everyone experiences it quite differently and there should be no rush. My experience has been that reassurance and outlining of a plan of investigation and action will provide much relief during this time. Generally, a woman will let me know when she is ready to proceed.

I have seen extreme bravery in the face of many losses. The willingness these families exhibit to press on deserves all the care and support a provider can give. I believe that many are able to go on because I don't give up on them; my commitment is a small token of support that all deserve. This more gentle approach includes making a plan of action so that the family will understand what to expect after the miscarriage is complete.

We discuss the workup for pregnancy loss and expectations for treatment, creating a timeline for future pregnancy. A few women prefer little intervention and are simply reassured by our discussion. After explaining that the results of an investigation may have a positive impact on their future pregnancy as well as their own health, most women are eager to do the required workup. It may come as a relief to learn whether there are certain familial conditions and genetic predispositions that may be the causes of early pregnancy losses, as well as medical conditions that may occur later in life, such as heart attack and stroke.

Chapter 4: Approaching Loss

A loss may not always require a D&C, but after 7-8 weeks it may be needed to prevent heavy bleeding and pain.

Larger fetuses need to be delivered and may not remain in utero for long periods of time due to the need to prevent DIC (disseminated intravascular coagulation).

A plan of action should be outlined and the family allowed to decide the level of investigation they desire.

Chapter 5

Thrombophilia

> Thrombophilia: A hypercoagulable condition, the genetic predisposition to form abnormal blood clots.

While there are a large number of complexities involved in pregnancy loss, thrombophilia seems to be the heart of the problem and is deserving of a chapter unto itself. Within our practice, 68% of the women presenting with pregnancy loss have some known form of thrombophilia. Understanding this has brought the incidence of loss in our practice to ~8%, in comparison to the national average of 25%.

Thrombophilia is not a disease, it is a genetic predisposition to have blood clots. It appears that 60-80% of the general population has some form of thrombophilia, some very mild, others severe. Given the proper circumstances, some of these thrombophilias may be expressed and may interfere with the establishment of a healthy pregnancy.

Pregnancy may be one of those special circumstances, which is itself a hypercoagulable state. This means that pregnant women are more at risk of having a blood clot. Even a tiny blood clot can block blood flow to the placenta and cause an early loss, or may simply restrict the flow as a baby grows, causing it to have intrauterine growth retardation. Taking birth control pills, hormonal replacement, or simply having a surgical procedure may also present a significant risk to having a heart attack, stroke, or pulmonary embolus.

The high percentage of people with thrombophilias may actually make it a norm, since the number one cause of death in the U.S. is cardiovascular disorders like heart attack, stroke, and pulmonary embolism. Yet in about 50% of the cases of thrombosis, the actual thrombophilias may not be found. This is likely due to our inability to test for every existing thrombosis. Fortunately, they are all treated in a similar way, so that in the instance of even a suspected tendency to clot, a provider has a number of ways to provide prophylaxis.

Preconception

Potential complications of thrombophilia may be divided into problems of preconception, complications during pregnancy, and postpartum and long-term challenges. Problems associated with preconception may be infertility and undiagnosed early pregnancy loss. When a couple is diagnosed with infertility, the woman may need to take fertility medications, which may be thrombogenic, putting her at risk for blood clots.

Pregnancy

During pregnancy, the expression of these genes varies from person to person, even within families. Not every pregnancy will be affected in the same way, and some may not be affected at all. The expression may also be affected by cofactors such as smoking, diet, and preexisting medical problems like high blood pressure. What seems to be predictable is that the expression of problems worsens as an individual ages. These genes tend to "turn on" when women reach their late 20s, and their effects seem to be more dramatic as time passes. This is the explanation I give to women who present having had recurrent losses that occur earlier and earlier with each subsequent pregnancy. For many women, the first may be at 10-12 weeks, the next at 8-10, and the last at 6 weeks or earlier. With each pregnancy, the woman is a bit older, and for some, it becomes much more difficult not only to carry a pregnancy, but also to become pregnant.

Complications may not be expressed the same way in every person with a particular clotting tendency, and it is virtually impossible to predict which type of problem may occur. This makes treatment more vital for a woman who has had a single loss. Waiting for a second or third loss makes no sense. The following may be a few of the potential complications associated with thrombophilia.

Ultra-early losses, also known as "chemical pregnancies" or "blighted ovum," appear to be common. Early signs of pregnancy, such as breast tenderness and missing a period for 1 or 2 days, are often present. Women often report "feeling pregnant," only to lose the feeling within a few days. HCG levels may rise slightly, although usually no higher than 25 miu. This, too, appears to be due to small clots at the site of implantation of the fertilized egg. The clotting process does not allow the egg to establish itself for growth in the womb.

However, even when the fetus survives the first trimester, these genes may present other problems. There are many concerns associated with thrombophilias, three of the most common being pregnancy-associated hypertension, intrauterine growth restriction, and oligohydramnios (low levels of amniotic fluid). These may manifest all together, or as single problems. When I encounter these problems, I begin my investigation by addressing the issues at hand, but always proceed to evaluate a patient's thrombophilias status. Increased fetal monitoring, bed rest, and hydration are my normal recommendations. If there is no improvement, or if the patient is noncompliant, hospitalization and IV hydration may be necessary.

First Trimester Loss

First trimester pregnancy loss lasts until 12 weeks gestation. With new ultrasound technology, it is possible to see a gestational sac as early as 5-6 weeks. A small fetus may be seen as early as 6 weeks. A miscarriage during this time may be marked by anything from no bleeding to spotting to heavy bleeding. Some losses are due to chromosomal anomalies, which are not compatible with life. Others appear to be due to thrombophilia. Often, this presents as what is termed a "missed abortion," where a fetal demise has occurred but the body takes weeks or months to begin the process of loss by bleeding. For instance, a patient whose fetal loss is discovered at 10 weeks with a fetal size of 7 weeks is often told that the fetus expired at 7 weeks. This may not be the case, but instead a manifestation of early growth restriction due to thrombophilia. The severe growth restriction may be present from the beginning of the pregnancy, with small clots in the placenta inhibiting the growth of the baby and ultimately ending in the demise.

Often, tissue obtained from a D&C will reveal fibrin deposits, which are associated with clot formation. Small-for-date measurements may also be seen prior to an actual loss in women with accurate menstrual dating and suspected thrombophilia. We give credence to our patients who are sure of their dates when an early sonogram lags behind those dates and a thrombophilia workup and close ultrasound observation and treatment is offered.

Finding thrombophilia or growth restriction begs the question of whether that pregnancy can be saved since the process had already begun. That is a decision between the patient, her family, and her healthcare provider. It is often a leap of faith for the patient who has not lost a pregnancy or had any other medical condition that warrants treatment for thrombophilia. The very least a provider can do is to inform the patient and provide her with thoughtful information in order to help her make a better decision for herself.

Second Trimester Loss

The end of week 12 starts the second trimester. During the second trimester, losses may occur with cervical incompetence, involving a premature rupture of membranes. A loss during this time also often appears to be evidence of a thrombophilia. When a loss occurs, the fetus and placenta are often complete and both large enough for separate pathologic evaluation. If a chromosomal anomaly is present, gross examination and chromosomal analysis may provide insight to the exact condition.

When the loss is due to a thrombophilia, the baby is often small, however no abnormalities are seen on a pathologic exam or autopsy.
The placenta may also be grossly small, and a microscopic exam often holds the answer to the demise. Often, the pathologist sees areas of infarction, or dead tissue, due to the failure of the blood supply. A large infarction may cause the ultimate demise. Another notation that may be seen is fibrin deposition, which is an indication of clot formation.

Third Trimester Loss

During the last trimester, women with pregnancy loss usually present with markedly decreased or absent fetal movements. The baby is again small in women with clotting tendencies. The placenta is small and areas of infarction may be seen with the naked eye, as well as by microscopic examination. Any unexplained second or third trimester loss is worthy of a thrombophilia workup.

Hypertension

Hypertension, or high blood pressure, tends to cause constriction of blood vessels and decreased blood flow through the umbilical cord and placenta. Hypertension in pregnancy may take many forms. Some women may present with a preexisting elevation of blood pressure, while others may develop elevations during the pregnancy, like preeclampsia and pregnancy induced hypertension. I evaluate all for thrombophilias.

It is common to see associated clotting tendencies, which can add to the decreased blood flow by causing clots that obstruct the blood flow to the placenta. When the blood flow is completely occluded, the area becomes infarcted, or dead. If enough of the placenta is infarcted, abnormalities in the fetal heart tracing may be evident. This may worsen in labor and increase the risk of cesarean for fetal distress. The combination of hypertension and thrombophilia may be lethal for the unborn. Treating both may optimize the outcome for the fetus.

Growth Restriction

Growth restriction is a very common problem where the size of the fetus lags behind the actual number of weeks pregnant. So a fetus of 30 actual weeks may only measure 28 weeks or less by sonogram or fundal height (the distance in centimeters from the top of the uterus to the top of the pubic bone is roughly equal to the number of weeks pregnant). Growth restriction occurs when there is a lack of adequate circulation of nutrition and oxygen to feed the growth of the baby. One may also see a restriction of growth due to certain viral illnesses, or with use of certain drugs.

This restriction leads to a small, malnourished baby who is often less resistant to the stress of labor. To increase perfusion I normally start with rest at home. This does not mean that a woman must be in bed at all times, just that she should not participate in the daily grind. Commuting to work, shopping, and engaging in housework are all discouraged. She may, however, engage her mind with work from home, prepare light meals for herself, and have visitors. Many of these women have some form of thrombophilia, and treatment with aspirin or Heparin may be started depending on the gestational age. Use of these medications and bed rest do not usually allow a baby to catch up in growth, although they may prevent a worsening of related problems.

There also appears to be a very early, but quite common form of growth restriction in the first trimester and early second trimester, which is often more devastating than those identified in the latter months. This may be because we have no way of easily detecting it. Even when a pregnancy has been established, fetal growth may lag behind the actual gestational age.

Women often present with menstrual dates suggesting an older fetus, however the ultrasound measurements may be smaller than expected. Unless a high index of suspicion is maintained, this discrepancy is most often attributed to incorrect dates. We normally inquire about the dates and history of menses, and date of conception or in vitro fertilization. If there is a discrepancy between the dates and the ultrasound, an ultrasound is repeated at a short interval of about two weeks to check the growth.

Oligohydramnios

Oligohydramnios is a common condition, affecting women with symptomatic thrombophilias in the third trimester. The amniotic fluid measured by ultrasound is low, representing another manifestation of poor placenta perfusion or blood flow. This may be caused by clots that partially obstruct blood from flowing to the fetus.

Oligohydramnios may also be seen in fetuses that have disorders of the urinary system and other non-thrombophilia related conditions. Bed rest and hydration may correct oligohydramnios, but in the most severe cases, delivery may be indicated if fetal movements become restricted.

Placental Abruption

Placental abruption is a premature separation of the placenta from the uterus. This acute event can occur at any time during pregnancy, and is most often associated with episodes of high blood pressure, although it may be seen as a result of trauma or infection. Placental abruption may cause fetal distress or even fetal death. If the separation is large enough, heavy bleeding in the area will follow. Blood clots then form in an attempt to prevent severe hemorrhage. If this condition is not immediately addressed, a massive clot will form and the clotting factors are quickly "used up" as the bleeding becomes uncontrollable. This condition is known as DIC, or disseminated intravascular coagulation. Hysterectomy may be indicated as a lifesaving measure for the mother.

Cerebral Palsy

Cerebral palsy (CP) is a condition that results in a spastic paralysis leading to mild to severe disabilities; the incidence of cerebral palsy in this country has remained largely unchanged since the 1960s, in spite of increased fetal monitoring, ultrasound, and cesarean sections. Obstetricians have long been scrutinized when a child was found to suffer from cerebral palsy. It is not often that this is a result of neglect on the part of the doctor or midwife (due to asphyxia, or lack of oxygen at the time of birth). A provider can perform perfectly and still have a delivery result in a child with CP. There is growing evidence that the events that result in cerebral palsy may occur in utero long before labor occurs.

These events may actually be a form of prenatal stroke, which can occur as early as the second trimester. When viewed side by side, children with cerebral palsy remarkably resemble people who have suffered a stroke. The prenatal stroke may be a result of decreased blood flow to the fetus due to partial infarction of the placenta. This decreases oxygen to the fetus, which may damage a vital part of the brain and result in paralysis of extremities and even mental retardation. These findings make diagnosis and treatment a vital part of preventive care for women with severe or complicated forms of thrombophilia.

Preterm Labor

Anticoagulant treatment may not be able to claim that it decreases preterm labor, yet I have noted that we have seen fewer cases of preterm labor among the patients we treat for thrombophilias. This may be a pleasant secondary effect of our increased vigilance in those patients, yet inflammation may be a cause of some preterm labor symptoms. This is evidenced by the efficacy of treating certain conditions with Heparin.

Inflammatory Process

What initiates the clotting process in the first place?

I believe that the clotting process may begin with an inflammation at the level of the lining of small blood capillaries. The inflammatory process may be due to injury to those blood vessels, perhaps during the process of implantation of the early embryo, called a blastocyst. Our bodies naturally heal the injury with our own multipotent stem cells, and no clotting process occurs.

However, if stem cells are not available or are inhibited by cofactors, the body will send the next best group of cells that fight infection and the inflammatory process—platelets and certain white blood cells. The clotting process then begins. When this occurs early in pregnancy, the placenta becomes clogged and the fetus expires. Later in pregnancy, the lack of flow may cause growth restriction and, when severe, may possibly cause cerebral palsy.

Another possible cause of the inflammatory process may be related to plasminogen, a protein found in the uterus, which is needed to degrade clots, as well as the membrane around the fertilized egg so that it can "hatch" in order for implantation to occur. The early embryo secretes plasminogen activator inhibitor (PAI), which prevents plasminogen from too much degradation or lytic activity. When PAI is too high, there is increased risk of clotting or thrombosis. PAI found in high amounts is also thought to prevent the hatching process, preventing implantation.

We have observed other possible associated complications of thrombophilia, such as those side effects of pulmonary embolism and deep venous thrombosis in pregnancy and during the postpartum period.

Abnormal PENTA Screens

Patients with thrombophilias may also have an abnormal PENTA screen, which is a second trimester test that measures blood levels of HCG, AFP, estriol and inhibin A. This test assesses the risk of having a pregnancy that may result in Down's syndrome, trisomy 18, or spina bifida. Although some improvements have been made to make this test more accurate, it still results in many heartbreaking false positive results.

The first problem with the test is that most patients do not understand that the results do not mean that the pregnancy will result in Down's syndrome, etc., but rather that the risk described in comparison to other women of the same age, race, and weight. When a family receives the news of a higher risk, the reaction is usually immediate panic. My experience with the PENTA screen is that while most results are "normal" and reassuring, the few that come back abnormal most often result in a baby without any problems.

However, perinatologists have long held that we should look for potential problems later in pregnancy, and should reassess at 28 weeks with ultrasound. What are some of the other possible problems that might arise at this juncture? Growth restriction, oligohydramnios, or other signs of fetal stress are very commonly cited.

It is my habit to test women with abnormal PENTA screens for thrombophilia. Not surprisingly, I have found that most of those tested have some form of genetic thrombophilia. These findings may explain the reasons for potential problems during the late second and third trimesters.

Another interesting note is that many patients with unusually high HCG levels at their initial visit also had abnormal PENTA screens between 16-20 weeks. Most of these patients had early ultrasounds to confirm viability between 6-10 weeks. Of the women who had high levels of HCG defined by >100,000 miu and sonograms at 6 weeks, many had two gestational sacs, or twins. A repeat ultrasound 2 weeks later often revealed a single fetus, however the elevated HCG level remains quite high. These high levels may

34

eventually result in false positive PENTA screens. The fact remains that the disappearing twin syndrome is another form of early pregnancy loss that should not be overlooked.

Ectopic Pregnancy

Ectopic pregnancies occur outside the uterus, the most common ectopic site being in the fallopian tube. Ectopic pregnancy is yet another form of early pregnancy loss. Most agree that injury to the fallopian tube, due to infection and endometriosis, is the major cause of this abnormality. We have seen a large number of women with no history of endometriosis, pelvic inflammatory disease, or other obvious diseases who suffer from ectopic pregnancies. In these cases, thrombophilia testing and treatment may be revealing.

Rising HCG levels in an early pregnancy, and/or microscopically damaged tubal lining cells, may call for repair involving white blood cells, which bring platelets responsible for clot formation in that same area.

Gestational Diabetes

Gestational diabetes is an inability to use the body's own insulin, resulting in elevated blood sugars. Diabetes can also cause problems with excessive amniotic fluid, larger fetuses, and a difficult birth process. Moreover, it may be associated with otherwise unexplained stillbirths. Gestational diabetes may be seen in women who have had previous insulin resistance problems, like polycystic ovarian syndrome, as well as in women who have never had a problem.

Chromosomal Disorders

Chromosomal disorders that influence pregnancy loss primarily include MTHFR and Factor V Leiden, among many others. Confounding these complications is the fact that there are thousands of genes yet to be discovered and catalogued. Knowing this, one would hardly believe that it is fairly easy to treat these problems. Yet this is true, and treatment should be limited only by patients' desires, rather than unwillingness on the behalf of the provider.

These predispositions do not go away, and they don't improve. Curiously enough, many believe that it is perfectly safe for people who have had previous thromboembolic events, like clots in the legs or lungs, not to take any preventive measures during pregnancy or when undergoing surgery.

Post-partum Complications

There are also potential complications that may occur after delivery. Pulmonary emboli, deep venous thrombosis, and septic pelvic thrombophlebitis are all problems that can affect a woman after her baby is born. Simple prevention is vital. Women must ambulate early after vaginal or cesarean births. It is also critical to consider cofactors such as obesity and smoking. Treatment with Heparin or even an oral anticoagulant like Coumadin may be needed (although Coumadin cannot be used during pregnancy as it crosses the placenta and affects the baby).

Long-term Complications

It is very important to note that knowledge of one's predispositions may prevent very serious future health problems that are not related to pregnancy.

Common Thrombophilia Classifications to Note

Homozygous: Having two of the same gene.

For instance, a patient with MTHFR may have two C677T genes. These patients may have more severe clotting tendencies that may occur earlier in life.

Heterozygous: Represents a single gene.

A woman who is heterozygous may have a solitary C677T or A1 gene. Although a pregnancy loss may occur, there may be only mild manifestations of thrombophilia.

In the case of complex heterozygosity, there are two different types of genes present, such as C677T and A1. For example, there are over 40 known mutations of the MTHFR gene.

Thrombophilia may be nature's method of population control, causing infertility and pregnancy loss in younger women, and stroke, heart attacks, and pulmonary emboli in older women. Other cofactors will certainly contribute to these problems, but recognition of the underlying genetic tendency to make clots is the key to prevention.

Prevention is the key to the problem. Unfortunately, most providers are trained to deal with the complications of thrombophilia rather than the prevention of those complications.

Providers must learn to change the paradigm. First, by considering any pregnancy loss worthy of investigation in order to prevent future losses. And second, by taking action to prevent future loss through treatment. Finally, they must give counsel and education on the long-term implications for the patient and their family.

Chapter 5: Thrombophilia

Thrombophilia is a genetic predisposition to blood clotting that may cause complications during pregnancy, and even fetal demise.

Physicians should take precautions to identify predispositions to thrombophilia and to prevent future loss through treatment, counseling, and education.

Chapter 6

Treatment Options for Thrombophilias

> A life saved is a statistic: a person hurt is an anecdote. Statistics are invisible: anecdotes are salient. Likewise, the risk of a Black Swan is invisible.
> — Nassim Nicholas Taleb —

Above all else, prevention is the key to successful pregnancy. Most patients and providers resist speaking in terms of prevention because it cannot be seen or measured. Doctors typically believe that if no bad outcome occurs then there is no reason to believe that there are any underlying problems with a patient, and no reason to expect any problems in the future.

As a result, medical practice is often a waiting game; wait until you have a problem, then try to deal with the damage. With a 25% rate of spontaneous pregnancy loss and 60-80% of people exhibiting a gene that may cause thrombophilia, why wait? There are many avenues of preventative treatment that can help avoid loss and unnecessary suffering.

Anticoagulants and Anti-inflammatories

Aspirin

My treatment regimen differs from patient to patient, and is dependent on multiple factors. There is no cookbook for thrombophilia treatment. Therapy with aspirin depends on the person, the thrombophilia type, and the individual's history. Aspirin, which comes from the humble willow bark, is an over-the-counter remedy effective for some clotting disorders. Aspirin may provide some protection in certain settings, and may be given when there are no obvious contraindications. It can be given preconceptually in infertility patients with proven antiphospholipid syndrome, or who are hetero- or homozygous for MTHFR, PAI, Protein S Protein C deficiency, Lipoprotein A, hyperhomocystenemia, and Factor V Leiden. There are also multiple other thrombophilias and autoimmune diseases that may be identified by a hematologist that can be treated with a simple dosage of aspirin (81 mg).

Generally, younger women (under 30) will respond well to aspirin alone. If the patient has suffered multiple losses or has had a personal history of clotting in her legs, a stroke, or a heart attack, I take into consideration her age, the kinds of losses, and the type of thrombophilia she has. Although aspirin may be an offering, I may ask her to entertain the possibility of taking a more potent anticoagulant.

If a patient is only on aspirin, I ask them to stop taking it at 36-37 weeks, as the possibility of delivery increases as one approaches term or 40 weeks. Aspirin therapy within two weeks of delivery may increase the chance of heavier than normal bleeding at the time of birth. This should be avoided when possible.

Aspirin Precautions

It has been said that if aspirin were to be brought to market as a new drug it would never obtain FDA approval due to its many potential uses and side effects. Above all, it is a potent anti-inflammatory and anticoagulant. As widely available as it is, aspirin should not be taken lightly, and usage should be discussed with your physician prior to starting the regimen. Patients are warned about easy bruising, prolonged bleeding with cut injuries, and gastrointestinal bleeding when ulcers are aggravated. Tinnitus, or ringing in the ears, may be associated with aspirin use. Aspirin is not recommended in women who are breast-feeding.

Heparin

Heparin is prescribed when there has been a pregnancy loss on aspirin alone, and in women with known histories of blood clots and certain thrombophilias as well as multiple losses. When previous, ultra-early losses or "chemical pregnancies" are suspected or confirmed, I often start Heparin prior to conception. This is introduced from ovulation through menses monthly. If a positive pregnancy test is confirmed, HCG levels are followed until an ultrasound is feasible.

Heparin is an injectable anticoagulant or blood thinner that aids in improving the flow of blood oxygen and nutrients to the growing fetus. It is injected under the skin to prevent the formation of blood clots in the major blood vessels of the mother and in the placenta. Although most people would prefer an oral anticoagulant like Coumadin, such medications are unsafe to take during pregnancy, as they cross the placental barrier. Depending on when it is given, Coumadin can cause severe developmental abnormalities, hemorrhaging, and even stillborns.

In contrast to Coumadin, Heparin does not cross the placental barrier, making it safe for use during pregnancy. In our practice, it is usually given in prophylactic dosing of 5000 units, twice daily. Most patients prefer the single dose of Lovenox to the mini dose of Heparin, however Heparin is more affordable and is covered by most insurers.

It is safe to use Heparin throughout the pregnancy, although patients should be examined vaginally from 35 weeks onward. Women are asked to hold their dose at term if they feel labor is imminent. This is done to prevent heavier than normal bleeding at the time of birth.

Heparin precautions are always taken. When therapy is initiated, weekly platelet counts are performed for the first month, with monthly counts thereafter. Most patients will use minidose Heparin, which does not increase the bleeding time, although can possibly cause a drop in platelet count. This is known as HIT, or Heparin induced thrombocytopenia.

HIT is a rare, but potentially devastating, complication. Although the platelet count is lowered, it appears that these cells are taken out of normal circulation and activated to cause increased clotting. This is why people with HIT have an increased risk of thrombosis, exactly the opposite of the desired effect of Heparin. Therefore, it is very important for anyone who develops a severe skin or allergic reaction while taking Heparin to seek immediate medical attention. It is not recommended to take Heparin if your provider is uncomfortable or unfamiliar with Heparin protocols. It is better to seek the advice of a hematologist or perinatologist, in addition to the primary provider.

Lovenox

Lovenox is a low molecular weight Heparin, which is longer acting than Heparin and therefore needs to be used only once a day when given in a prophylactic dose. I usually prescribe this to women who have had more than one loss, or have had a failure on aspirin alone. Women over 35 with a known thrombophilia, multiple losses, or suspected ultra early losses often benefit from prophylactic dosing. Those who require higher dosing often may have had a thromboembolic event during pregnancy or have multiple thrombophilias. A hematology consult is necessary for proper dosing. We follow these patients with Anti Xa levels monthly and platelets weekly for 4 weeks, and then monthly for the rest of the pregnancy.

Lovenox can be used for the first trimester until approximately 35 or 36 weeks gestation. At that time, a change is made to Heparin. The change is made due to the potential risk of epidural hematoma in patients on Lovenox who receive a labor epidural. An epidural hematoma can lead to severe headache and difficulty walking, numbness, and speech problems. Lovenox may be restarted the day after delivery to prevent postpartum blood clotting in the mother.

Combination therapy is more controversial and may create greater risk of bleeding. This method involves using Heparin or Lovenox in addition to aspirin. This is used when a single therapy, with Lovenox or Heparin given from ovulation to menses, has not been effective to prevent loss. The combination may be the only effective method for some patients. The process first begins by decreasing the initial inflammatory response to implantation of the fertilized egg with aspirin, and then allowing blood flow to the embryo with Lovenox. I usually reserve this combination for women who have a very poor obstetrical history and are over the age of 39 or 40.

FAQ Regarding Anticoagulants and Anti-inflammatories

Will treatment for thrombophilia make me carry a pregnancy with major abnormalities to term?

No.

Moreover, many women who have never been treated and have a presumably "normal" pregnancy will deliver a full term infant with congenital abnormalities. This will occur in about 7% of all pregnancies, regardless of medications taken for treatment of thrombophilia.

Why must I stop taking Lovenox or Heparin prior to delivery?

Theoretically, there is no good obstetrical reason to stop, since prophylactic doses of Heparin should not increase the bleeding time. We do, however, suggest stopping the medication because anesthesiologists are concerned about the risk of epidural hematoma in women who receive that form of pain management.

Hormonal Therapy

Progesterone is a hormone that may be given to help support the lining of the uterus in women who may have hormonal imbalances such as luteal phase defects. It is usually continued throughout the first trimester until 12 weeks, giving the placenta time to begin its own production of progesterone. A low progesterone level during early pregnancy is often evidence of a non-viable fetus or poor ultimate prognosis. Although I do perform progesterone hormone treatment if low progesterone levels are documented, I have not found that adding progesterone alone will improve future pregnancy outcomes. It is unclear whether the low levels of progesterone cause the demise, or if a drop in hormone levels follows the demise. In addition, some progestins may be thrombogenic and may contribute to clot formation in women with thrombophilia. This makes it particularly important to treat any underlying thrombophilia.

Vitamin Therapy

Folate

Folate is extremely important during pregnancy, as it is necessary for the production of DNA, and for DNA replication. A deficiency may hinder cell division at a time when it is needed most, when the embryonic cells and stem cells are proliferating. This may particularly affect the small blood vessel forming between the placenta and the wall of the uterus. There are even studies that suggest an increased risk of Down's syndrome, or trisomy 21, in women with abnormalities of folate.

B12

B12 is needed for DNA synthesis in the fetus. Vitamin absorption may be problematic for some women, in which case B12 injections can be administered.

Vitamin D

There is some evidence that low levels of Vitamin D may cause mood disorders, as well as an increased risk for preeclampsia, the high blood pressure of pregnancy. Vitamin D levels should be checked when the patient presents for prenatal care.

Monitoring Regimens

How do monitoring regimens help? The aim of monitoring the progress of pregnancy in those with thrombophilia is prevention. The prevention of the many potential complications related to thrombophilia is outlined in Chapter 5. The following case study offers a nice example of how close observation may prevent a potentially lethal outcome.

A 32 year-old patient with one previous normal pregnancy and no personal or family history of thrombophilia came to see me 5 years ago. She had an uncomplicated pregnancy until approximately 28 weeks, at which time she developed elevated blood pressure. Lab testing for preeclampsia was negative, and she was placed on bed rest at home, treated with medication for her blood pressure, and tested for thrombophilia. Additionally, she was asked to have weekly biophysical profiles (see below). The patient's biophysical profile was normal at 10 out of 10, however Doppler studies (see below) showed an extremely high resistance to blood flow at the level of the umbilical cord, and very low resistance to flow at the level of the brain.

She was immediately sent to the perinatologist, who concurred with our evaluation. She was admitted to a tertiary care center with a neonatal ICU and given steroids to mature the fetal lungs. She delivered the baby the following day after developing a severe, atypical preeclampsia. The baby and mother both did very well in the birth. This course of monitoring allowed us a small window of opportunity to treat both effectively. Had we simply relied on biophysical scores and her lab work, she would have been sent home on bed rest, and possibly have delivered a stillborn and/or had severe complications herself.

Biophysical Profile

A biophysical profile is a prenatal test that is widely used to evaluate fetal well-being. It is a test that looks at:

>Fetal breathing motions.
>Fetal movement.
>Fetal tone of limbs.
>Amniotic fluid volume.
>Fetal heart rate.

A score is then given based on each measurement, from 0 to 10. A score of 8 to 10 out of 10 is considered reassuring, while 6 out of 10 or below requires further evaluation.

Antepartum testing provides a window of opportunity for prevention or worsening of certain obstetrical complications.

Doppler Studies

A growth ultrasound is typically done when a provider suspects a smaller or larger growth of the fetus. Fetuses showing signs of poor growth may be seen in thrombophilia, in smokers, and in other conditions that affect the blood flow.

Umbilical Doppler is an ultrasound study of the resistance of blood through the umbilical cord of growing fetuses. Generally, we expect a fairly low resistance to flow. Certain conditions may cause a relative restriction of blood flow. Examples of these conditions would be hypertension and thrombophilia.

Along with middle cerebral artery Dopplers, these studies may detect subtle problems with blood flow in advance of potentially devastating problems. A middle cerebral artery Doppler is an ultrasound study of the resistance of blood flow through an artery in the brain of the fetus.

Perinatologists serve as high-risk pregnancy specialists, and are usually consulted if the patient will be over 35 at the time of pregnancy, or if they have medical conditions like heart disease.

A hematologist, or blood disorder specialist, may be called upon to act as a consultant during preconception, pregnancy, and in the postpartum period. They may order additional testing if needed, and interpret the results of the Anti X1a levels and platelets in order to adjust Lovenox and Heparin levels when needed.

Understanding treatment options for thrombophilias can transform and empower a patient and the course of her own and her family's life.

Chapter 6: Treatment Options for Thrombophilias

Treatment options for thrombophilias include:

- Anticoagulant and Anti-inflammatory Treatments

- Hormone Therapy

- Vitamin Therapy

- Monitoring Regimes

Chapter 7

Freedom of Choice

> My basic principle is that you don't make decisions because they
> are easy; you don't make them because they are cheap; you don't
> make them because they're popular; you make them because
> they're right.
> — Theodore Hesburgh —

I am passionate about offering choices. As such, our office often attracts
couples that are seeking alternatives to the "traditional" non-investigation
of pregnancy loss. Their stories may vary, but their complaints are often in
the same vein. Most of all, they want to be heard and they want something
done to remove their sense of helplessness.

Most have been told to wait or just to try again. Many are angry because
they are aware of possible investigations that could have been done but
were deemed unnecessary. I hope the previous chapters have explained the
necessity for such investigations, and their positive, long-lasting
implications for both the individual and their families.

Unfortunately, insurance companies continue to thwart the efforts of many
families by refusing to cover certain tests or medications. This sends the
detrimental message that their clientele should stay healthy or die, have a
healthy baby or not bother. They cite articles and studies to defend their
positions and act contrary to the desires of the patients and their providers.
I understand cost-saving measures, however preventive measures taken
may save even more money as opposed to the repercussions of unfortunate
medical oversights.

Of course, it is ultimately your choice as a patient to find a way to get what
you need most—starting with being informed about your own medical
history, reproductive health, and risk for pregnancy loss. Most doctors are
aware of alternative methods of diagnosis and treatment, but may not offer
them to their patients because they are also aware that the insurers will not

pay for these methods. As a patient, you have the ability (and responsibility) to decide to what lengths you will go for your own health. One must remember that the patient may pay for tests and treatments, and later file appeals to cover costs. The most critical gifts I can offer my patients are options for their care.

Most women who present after a miscarriage want answers to their unanswered questions, such as: *Did I do something to cause this? Did I exercise too much, or was it caused by intimacy? Will I ever be able to have a baby?*

As a physician, I do not claim to know all the answers, but I do always sit with the family and listen to their concerns. This process is equally valuable for me, because I, too, wonder what I could have done to make it a better pregnancy. Often, it is much harder for me to explain why a person should take a certain medicine as opposed to simply urging them to "try again". Such platitudes take much less time, and would not implicate me in the loss prevention process.

Yet the only currency I have to work with is my knowledge base, and the time I spend with my patients. I feel it is both my duty and privilege to offer the full power of these tools to each woman I treat.

Ultimately, I am committed to treating the distinct needs of each woman who enters my office, and am honored to practice medicine in this way.

Chapter 7: Freedom of Choice
Each woman is responsible for seizing control of her own reproductive health and pregnancy process, despite challenges posed by the medical establishment.
Each healthcare provider is equally responsible for seeking to provide the best, most individualized care and consult possible to every patient.

Conclusion

The Future is Prevention

The order of the universe is toward compassion.
— Pete Terpenning —

I have a rather lofty aspiration when it comes to my patients, and all people in the world: For each to live a long and fruitful life, and when it is time to die, to go peacefully in their sleep and never suffer. Yet whether one has a pregnancy loss as a younger woman, or experiences a loss of ability through stroke later in life, suffering seems to be the one constant in human experience.

The compassionate medical provider cannot cure all illness or prevent death. Medical practitioners must learn to understand the ways in which prevention is directly related to quality of life. When medical problems are allowed to reoccur without being addressed, all aspects of the patient's life are affected.

Medicine has always been guided by observation and comparisons of treatment options for diseases that have already occurred. Essentially, a medical provider's living is earned from the sickness and suffering of their patients. Yet new demand is slowly turning us toward prevention. This will become increasingly important as humans live longer. People are not seeking to live longer only to suffer the ravages of preventable disease, but to live fuller, healthier, and more productive lives.

For many women, prevention is an easy next step as they present after having a miscarriage. We can then test and treat their subsequent pregnancies, advise them about the risks to their family members, and discuss how to avoid clotting problems in the future. It is easier for them because they are highly motivated. Once successful, we have an obligation to uphold continued vigilance against potential future medical problems.

It is important to remember that thrombophilia is not a disease state; on the contrary, it is a key to prevention and understanding. A predisposition to thrombophilia cuts away the excuses people have regarding their family histories, like guessing at associated causes of heart attack, obesity, or a myriad of other morbidities. While cofactors such as smoking, lack of exercise, and many others no doubt contribute to early death, genetic makeup provides a very simple explanation—one was made that way.

If one understands how they are made, specific risks to that individual become clear, and it is possible to take the necessary behavioral precautions, medications, and procedures for health. For example, a healthy, active postmenopausal woman may not be so interested in hormonal replacement if it is found that she has a thrombophilia that puts her at a higher risk for stroke or heart attack. This is a question a woman with thrombophilia will face in the next chapter of her life after having children.

While prevention is critical, physicians and patients tend to eschew it because there is no way to prove the positive effects of prevention (since nothing—but health—occurs). The key to proving prevention, then, is patience. Evidence-based medicine has its place, but it should not replace a provider's ability to take a step back from an individual patient and think about what is best for that person.

Evidence-based medicine does not always provide for individuals, and may not always look at a problem in the correct way. This reaffirms the importance of refusing to rest on the merits of one or two treatment modalities, and of continually seeking out potential options.

Through thrombophilia identification and patient education, we come one step closer to the goal of using prevention to live longer and healthier lives. When families ask about other long-term risk implications of thrombophilia, I advise that their risks outside of pregnancy may be heart attack, stroke, deep venous thrombosis, and with certain thrombophilias, an increased risk of colon and unusual cancers, like lung cancer in non-smokers. This knowledge is not meant to frighten anyone, but is instead meant to help guide and support future health.

It does not take a medical doctor to look at a strong family history of heart attack to know that an individual in that family is at high risk. In the same way, no formal medical training is needed to look at someone who is obese, diabetic, and hypertensive to understand the risk of life-changing complications. A patient-provider partnership founded upon education regarding the individual's potential risks may avoid or minimize this undesirable outcome.

To this, I ask simply, why suffer?

Society today is more concerned than ever with the rights women hold to make decisions about their own bodies. There are many, doctors included, who seek to dictate a woman's ability to choose the outcome of her pregnancy. Yet an equally critical issue is the woman's right to know and do everything she possibly can to ensure the prevention of pregnancy complications, and the maintenance of early fetal life. In this regard, a willing determination, an openness to learning, and a competent medical care provider are her strongest tools for success.

Conclusion: The Future is Prevention

Medicine is dynamic, changing every day by necessity.

There is no room in healthcare for the attitude that "everything" has been done.

Your genetic predispositions do not change, making prevention practices imperative to future health.

Glossary

Anencephalic - A birth defect caused by the lack of closure of the neural tube in a developing fetus, resulting in the absence of formation of parts of the scalp, skull, and fetal brain.

Cerebral Palsy - A birth defect caused by damage to the developing fetal brain, resulting in spasticity and problems with movement.

Coumadin - An oral anticoagulant, or blood thinner, **not** for use during pregnancy.

Deep venous thrombosis - A blood clot in deep veins, typically in the lower legs.

D&C - Dilation and curettage is a surgical procedure in which the cervix is dilated and tissue is removed from the uterus.

DIC - Disseminated intravascular coagulation is a disorder that "consumes" all of the body's clotting factors, resulting in uncontrolled bleeding.

Factor V Leiden - An inherited type of thrombophilia, or tendency to form clots.

Folic Acid - Also known as folate, and is vitamin B9.

Heparin - An injectable anticoagulant, or blood thinner, which aids in the prevention and extension of blood clots.

Heterozygous - Having two different genes.

HCG - Human chorionic gonadotropin is a chemical measured in both urine and blood pregnancy tests.

HIT - Heparin induced thrombocytopenia, a complication of taking Heparin. HIT results in an abnormal drop in blood platelet levels.

Homozygous - Having two of the same genes.

Hyperhomocystenemia - An unusual elevation of homocysteine, which may be associated with the abnormal formation of blood clots.

Hypertension - High blood pressure.

Hysterosalpingogram - An x-ray study of the uterus and fallopian tubes to look for tubal blockage and abnormalities of the uterus.

Intrauterine growth restriction - Also known as intrauterine growth retardation. Indicates a limitation of fetal growth due to problems of the umbilical cord and/or placenta.

LEEP procedure - Loop Electrical Excision Procedure, used to remove abnormal or precancerous tissue from the cervix.

Level II ultrasound - A sonogram performed by a perinatologist or maternal fetal medicine specialist.

Lovenox - An injectable anticoagulant, or blood thinner, which aids in the prevention and extension of blood clots.

MTHFR - Methylenetetrahydrofolate reductase is an inherited type of thrombophilia, or tendency to form clots.

Oligohydramnios - Abnormally low amniotic fluid.

PENTA screen - Second trimester maternal serum screen, used to detect certain genetic problems such as Down's syndrome.

Placental abruption - Abnormal separation of the placenta from the uterine wall prior to birth.

Plasminogen Activator Inhibitor - Inhibits the breakdown of blood clots. May also prevent implantation of the fertilized egg.

Preeclampsia - High blood pressure during pregnancy, marked by abnormal swelling, headache, changes in vision, and elevated urine proteins.

Protein S Protein C Deficiency - The lack of proteins that regulate clot formation and inflammation.

Pulmonary embolus - A blood clot in the blood vessels of one or both lungs, which prevents oxygen exchange. When the clot is large enough, the person will die due to the inability to breathe.

Quad Screen - An older, second trimester maternal serum screen used to detect certain genetic problems such as Down's syndrome.

Sonohysterogram - An ultrasound using saline to evaluate the uterine lining.

Thrombophilia - The genetic predisposition to form abnormal blood clots.

Acknowledgments

I want to offer my profound thanks to:

Mommy, for everything;

My sister, for a wonderful title;

My family and friends, for all of their love and support;

The NIH, for statistics on maternal mortality;

And last but not least, to Lily at Ivy Eyes Editing, for your guidance and patience on the path of book publishing.

Made in the USA
Columbia, SC
20 March 2018